THE OSTEOPOROSIS TREATMENT HANDBOOK

BUILDING BSTRONG BONES

AMANDA FERDINAND

Copyright

Table of Contents

INTRODUCTION

Osteoporosis is a progressive skeletal disorder characterized by decreased bone mass and deterioration of bone microarchitecture, leading to increased fragility and susceptibility to fractures. It is a major global public health concern, particularly affecting postmenopausal women and the elderly population. As life expectancy rises, the prevalence of osteoporosis is expected to increase, posing significant challenges to healthcare systems worldwide. Fractures resulting from osteoporosis, especially hip and vertebral fractures, are associated with substantial morbidity, reduced quality of life, loss of independence, and increased mortality. Therefore, effective management strategies are essential not only to treat but also to prevent the disease and its complications.

The management of osteoporosis involves a comprehensive and multifaceted approach, targeting both the reduction of fracture risk and the improvement of bone health. Central to this is the identification of individuals at risk through clinical assessment and diagnostic tools such as bone mineral density (BMD) testing using dual-energy X-ray absorptiometry (DEXA). Early diagnosis enables timely intervention, which can significantly alter the course of the disease.

Therapeutic strategies encompass lifestyle modifications, pharmacological treatments, and fall prevention. Lifestyle measures, including adequate intake of calcium and vitamin D, regular weight-bearing and muscle-strengthening exercise, smoking cessation, and limiting alcohol consumption, play a foundational role in maintaining bone health. Pharmacologic interventions, such as bisphosphonates, selective estrogen receptor modulators (SERMs), parathyroid hormone analogs, and monoclonal antibodies like denosumab, have proven effective in increasing bone density and reducing fracture risk. The choice of therapy is often guided by the severity of bone loss, patient-specific factors, and risk-benefit considerations.

In addition to treatment, secondary prevention strategies are critical, especially for individuals who have already sustained a fragility fracture. This includes coordinated care models such as fracture liaison services (FLS) that ensure appropriate post-fracture assessment and treatment to prevent recurrence.

Effective osteoporosis management requires a collaborative, patient-centered approach involving primary care physicians, endocrinologists, rheumatologists, physical therapists, and nutritionists. Patient education and adherence to therapy are also vital components of successful long-term management. In summary, managing osteoporosis involves not only treating the existing condition but also implementing preventive measures to reduce future fracture risk. With early detection, individualized treatment plans, and ongoing patient engagement, the burden of osteoporosis can be significantly mitigated, leading to improved patient outcomes and enhanced quality of life.

CHAPTER 1

UNDERSTANDING OSTEOPOROSIS

Osteoporosis is a chronic, progressive skeletal disorder characterized by low bone mass and deterioration of bone microarchitecture, leading to increased bone fragility and susceptibility to fractures. Often referred to as the "silent disease," osteoporosis progresses without symptoms until a fracture occurs, typically in the hip, spine, or wrist. With the aging global population, osteoporosis is rapidly emerging as a significant public health concern due to its associated morbidity, mortality, and healthcare costs. Understanding the underlying mechanisms and epidemiological trends of this disease is crucial for effective prevention, diagnosis, and management.

DEFINING OSTEOPOROSIS

The World Health Organization (WHO) defines osteoporosis based on bone mineral density (BMD) measurements. A T-score (which compares a patient's BMD to that of a healthy

30-year-old adult) of -2.5 or lower indicates osteoporosis. A T-score between -1.0 and -2.5 is considered osteopenia, a condition of low bone mass that precedes osteoporosis. Osteoporosis can be broadly categorized into:

- **Primary osteoporosis**: Commonly age-related or postmenopausal, occurring without an underlying disease.
- Secondary osteoporosis: Results from medical conditions, medications, or lifestyle factors that disrupt bone remodeling.

BONE BIOLOGY AND REMODELING

Bone Structure

- Bones are dynamic organs made up of a matrix composed of collagen and mineral (primarily hydroxyapatite). The skeletal system serves structural, metabolic, and hematopoietic functions. Bone strength is determined by bone density and bone quality, including microarchitecture, turnover, and mineralization.

Bone Remodeling Process

Bone remodeling is a lifelong process that maintains skeletal integrity by replacing old bone with new tissue. It involves the coordinated activity of:

- Osteoclasts – cells that resorb (break down) bone.
- Osteoblasts – cells that form new bone.
- Osteocytes – mature bone cells involved in signaling and maintenance.

This remodeling is regulated by systemic hormones (e.g., estrogen, parathyroid hormone, calcitonin), local cytokines, and mechanical stress. In osteoporosis, there is an imbalance in remodeling where bone resorption outpaces bone formation, leading to net bone loss.

PATHOPHYSIOLOGY OF OSTEOPOROSIS

Estrogen Deficiency

- One of the most significant contributors to postmenopausal osteoporosis is estrogen deficiency. Estrogen inhibits osteoclast-mediated bone resorption. Its decline during menopause leads to increased osteoclast activity, enhanced bone turnover, and accelerated bone loss, particularly in trabecular (spongy) bone.

Aging

- Aging contributes to both reduced bone formation and increased bone resorption. Age-related decline in osteoblast function and increased oxidative stress impact bone quality. In addition, calcium absorption from the gut decreases, and renal calcium conservation is impaired with age.

Calcium and Vitamin D Deficiency

- Calcium is essential for bone mineralization, and vitamin D facilitates calcium absorption and bone remodeling. Deficiencies in either result in secondary hyperparathyroidism, stimulating bone resorption and accelerating bone loss.

Chronic Inflammation and Oxidative Stress

- Chronic inflammation and oxidative stress can stimulate osteoclastogenesis via cytokines such as IL-1, IL-6, and TNF-alpha. This is particularly relevant in chronic conditions such as rheumatoid arthritis and inflammatory bowel disease, which are associated with secondary osteoporosis.

TYPES OF OSTEOPOROSIS

Postmenopausal Osteoporosis (Type I)
- This type affects women within 15-20 years after menopause. It predominantly involves trabecular bone, leading to vertebral compression fractures and distal forearm fractures.

Senile Osteoporosis (Type II)
- Typically occurs after age 70 in both sexes. It involves both trabecular and cortical bone, leading to hip and pelvic fractures. Age-related hormonal changes, nutritional deficiencies, and decreased physical activity contribute to this form.

Secondary Osteoporosis

Secondary osteoporosis is due to identifiable causes such as:
- Endocrine disorders (e.g., hyperthyroidism, Cushing's syndrome)
- Gastrointestinal disorders (e.g., celiac disease, malabsorption)
- Hematologic and autoimmune diseases

- Medications: glucocorticoids, anticonvulsants, chemotherapy, proton pump inhibitors
- Lifestyle factors: smoking, alcohol abuse, low physical activity

EPIDEMIOLOGY OF OSTEOPOROSIS

Global Prevalence

- According to the International Osteoporosis Foundation, more than 200 million people worldwide are affected by osteoporosis. One in three women and one in five men over the age of 50 will experience osteoporotic fractures in their lifetime.

Demographic Differences

- Gender: Women are at higher risk due to lower peak bone mass and hormonal changes after menopause. However, men have a higher morbidity and mortality rate after osteoporotic fractures.
- Age: Risk increases significantly with age due to cumulative bone loss and higher fall risk.
- Ethnicity: Caucasian and Asian populations have a higher risk compared

to African populations. However, fracture rates are rising globally due to aging populations and changing lifestyles.

Fracture Burden

- Hip fractures are the most serious, often leading to long-term disability or death. Vertebral fractures are also common but frequently go undiagnosed, contributing to chronic pain and deformity. Wrist fractures are more common in early osteoporosis and often serve as a sentinel event.

Economic Impact

- Osteoporosis imposes a substantial economic burden. In the United States alone, the annual cost of osteoporotic fractures exceeds $20 billion. Costs include acute care, long-term rehabilitation, and lost productivity. As the population ages, this burden is projected to rise significantly.

RISK FACTORS FOR OSTEOPOROSIS

Non-Modifiable Risk Factors

- Age: Bone mass peaks by the third decade and declines thereafter.

- Sex: Females, especially postmenopausal, are more susceptible.
- Family history: Genetic predisposition plays a role in peak bone mass and bone loss rates.
- Ethnicity: Higher risk in Caucasians and Asians.

Modifiable Risk Factors

- Nutritional deficiencies: Low intake of calcium, vitamin D, and protein
- Sedentary lifestyle: Lack of weight-bearing and resistance exercises
- Smoking: Interferes with calcium absorption and bone formation
- Alcohol: Excessive intake impairs bone metabolism
- Low body weight: Associated with reduced bone mass

SILENT NATURE OF THE DISEASE

- One of the challenges in managing osteoporosis is its asymptomatic nature until a fracture occurs. Loss of height, kyphosis, and back pain may be the first signs, often too late to prevent severe damage. This underscores the importance of early screening and risk assessment in at-risk populations.

Bone Density and Diagnosis

- Although the focus of this chapter is pathophysiology and epidemiology, a brief understanding of diagnosis enhances the context.

Bone Mineral Density (BMD): The gold standard for diagnosis is dual-energy X-ray absorptiometry (DEXA), which measures BMD and provides a T-score. The WHO criteria are:

- Normal: T-score ≥ -1.0

- Osteopenia: T-score between -1.0 and -2.5

- Osteoporosis: T-score ≤ -2.5

- Severe osteoporosis: T-score ≤ -2.5 with one or more fragility fractures

PREVENTIVE IMPLICATIONS OF EPIDEMIOLOGICAL TRENDS

- The rising global incidence of osteoporosis and related fractures presents a call to action for public health systems. Given the long asymptomatic phase, population-wide measures such as public education, early screening, and lifestyle interventions are critical.

Global Health Initiatives

- Organizations like the International Osteoporosis Foundation and National Osteoporosis Foundation promote awareness campaigns, research funding, and preventive health policies.

Key public health recommendations include:

- Calcium and vitamin D supplementation in at-risk groups
- Promotion of physical activity
- Fall prevention strategies
- Screening programs for early detection
- Fracture liaison services for secondary prevention

Future Perspectives and Research

Recent advances in molecular biology and genetics are deepening our understanding of bone metabolism. Novel markers for bone turnover, genetic profiling for risk prediction, and targeted biological therapies (e.g., sclerostin inhibitors) are emerging.

Ongoing research is also exploring:

- Gut microbiota and its impact on bone health
- Role of oxidative stress and mitochondrial dysfunction
- Digital tools and AI-driven algorithms for fracture risk prediction
- Telemedicine for remote screening and patient education

Osteoporosis represents a major and growing health burden worldwide, driven by an aging population and sedentary lifestyles. It is a complex condition rooted in hormonal, nutritional, mechanical, and genetic factors. The disease progresses silently but culminates in devastating fractures that significantly impair quality of life and increase mortality.

Understanding the pathophysiology and epidemiological dynamics of osteoporosis is the foundation for effective prevention and management. A proactive approach—through risk factor modification, early diagnosis, and comprehensive care—can substantially reduce the human and economic toll of this condition.

As we deepen our knowledge and refine our strategies, interdisciplinary collaboration and public awareness will remain central to combating this silent epidemic and improving the bone health of future generations.

CHAPTER 2

RISK FACTORS AND CAUSES

Osteoporosis is often dubbed the "silent thief" because it gradually erodes bone density without producing overt symptoms until a fracture occurs. While it is typically associated with aging, especially in postmenopausal women, a wide array of factors—both intrinsic and extrinsic—contribute to its development. Understanding the risk factors and causes of osteoporosis is essential for early identification, preventive strategies, and individualized care plans. This chapter delves into the multifactorial etiology of osteoporosis, categorizing the risk factors into non-modifiable, modifiable, and secondary causes, and explores their impact on bone health across various populations.

NON-MODIFIABLE RISK FACTORS

1. Age

- Aging is the most significant non-modifiable risk factor for osteoporosis. Bone mass peaks by the third decade of life, and after the age of 35, bone resorption begins to exceed bone formation, leading to gradual bone loss. This age-related decline accelerates further in older adults due to decreased osteoblast function, hormonal changes, reduced physical activity, and poor nutritional absorption.

2. Sex

Women are at a markedly higher risk than men for osteoporosis. This is largely due to:

- Lower peak bone mass in females compared to males.
- Menopause and the accompanying estrogen deficiency, which accelerates bone loss.
- Longer life expectancy in women increases the window for developing age-related osteoporosis.
- However, men are not immune. Though osteoporosis is underdiagnosed in males, they suffer greater morbidity and

mortality following osteoporotic fractures, particularly hip fractures.

3. Ethnicity and Race

- Caucasian and Asian populations are more likely to develop osteoporosis compared to African and Hispanic populations. This may be due to differences in skeletal structure, bone turnover rates, lifestyle factors, and genetic predispositions. African Americans tend to have higher peak bone mass and thicker cortical bones, offering some protective advantage.

4. Genetics and Family History

- Genetic factors account for up to 80% of peak bone mass. A family history of osteoporosis or fragility fractures, particularly hip fractures in a parent, significantly increases the risk. Specific genes related to vitamin D receptor activity, collagen formation, and estrogen metabolism may influence individual susceptibility.

MODIFIABLE RISK FACTORS

1. Nutrition

- **Calcium Deficiency:** Calcium is critical for bone mineralization. Inadequate intake leads to decreased bone density and can trigger secondary hyperparathyroidism, which accelerates bone resorption.
- **Vitamin D Deficiency:** Vitamin D enhances intestinal calcium absorption. Deficiency reduces calcium uptake, promotes bone loss, and increases fall risk due to muscle weakness. Populations at risk include older adults, individuals with limited sun exposure, darker skin pigmentation, or those with malabsorption syndromes.
- **Protein Deficiency:** Adequate protein is necessary for bone matrix formation and muscle strength. Malnutrition, particularly in the elderly, compromises skeletal integrity and increases fall and fracture risks.
- **Excessive Salt, Caffeine, and Phosphorus:** High sodium intake promotes urinary calcium loss. Excessive caffeine and carbonated drinks containing phosphoric acid may interfere

with calcium metabolism, although these effects are modest when calcium intake is adequate.

2. Physical Inactivity

- Weight-bearing and resistance exercises stimulate bone remodeling. Sedentary lifestyles lead to lower bone mass, muscle atrophy, and increased risk of falls. Mechanical loading from physical activity is essential for maintaining bone strength and structural integrity.

3. Smoking

- Cigarette smoking impairs osteoblast activity, reduces intestinal calcium absorption, lowers estrogen levels, and induces early menopause. Smokers have a significantly higher risk of fractures than non-smokers.

4. Alcohol Consumption

- Excessive alcohol intake disrupts bone remodeling by inhibiting osteoblast function and enhancing bone resorption. It also contributes to poor nutrition, increases fall risk, and can result in secondary liver disease affecting vitamin D metabolism.

5. Low Body Weight or BMI

- A body mass index (BMI) below 18.5 is a well-established risk factor for osteoporosis. Lower body weight is associated with decreased mechanical stress on bones, lower estrogen levels, and reduced fat stores that contribute to estrogen production. Underweight individuals also tend to have poorer nutritional reserves.

SECONDARY CAUSES OF OSTEOPOROSIS

Secondary osteoporosis results from identifiable medical conditions or medication use that interfere with bone remodeling. Recognizing and managing these underlying causes is vital to preventing further bone loss.

1. Endocrine Disorders

- **Hyperthyroidism**: Excess thyroid hormone accelerates bone turnover, leading to net bone loss. Overtreatment with levothyroxine can induce iatrogenic hyperthyroidism and contribute to osteoporosis.

- **Hyperparathyroidism:** Primary hyperparathyroidism causes elevated parathyroid hormone (PTH) levels, stimulating osteoclasts and increasing bone resorption, especially in cortical bone.
- **Cushing's Syndrome:** Excess cortisol (endogenous or exogenous) inhibits osteoblast activity, increases osteoclast survival, and promotes bone resorption. Chronic glucocorticoid exposure is a major cause of secondary osteoporosis.
- **Diabetes Mellitus:** Both Type 1 and Type 2 diabetes are associated with increased fracture risk. Type 1 diabetics tend to have low bone mass, while Type 2 patients may have normal or increased bone mass but poorer bone quality due to glycation and microvascular complications.
- **Hypogonadism:** In men, reduced testosterone levels impair bone formation and maintenance. Hypogonadism may result from aging, chronic illness, or medical treatment such as androgen deprivation therapy for prostate cancer.

2. Gastrointestinal Disorders

- Conditions that impair nutrient absorption directly impact bone health.
- Celiac disease and inflammatory bowel disease (IBD) reduce calcium and vitamin D absorption and are associated with systemic inflammation that exacerbates bone loss.
- Chronic liver disease interferes with vitamin D metabolism and impairs bone matrix production.
- Gastric bypass surgery (especially Roux-en-Y) affects calcium absorption and increases fracture risk.

RHEUMATOLOGIC AUTOIMMUNE DISEASES

a. Rheumatoid Arthritis (RA)

- RA is a chronic inflammatory disease associated with systemic bone loss, due to the combined effects of inflammatory cytokines (e.g., TNF-α), corticosteroid use, reduced mobility, and poor nutrition.

b. Systemic Lupus Erythematosus (SLE)

- SLE patients often experience osteoporosis from chronic inflammation, corticosteroid therapy, and decreased sun exposure leading to vitamin D deficiency.

Chronic Kidney Disease (CKD)

- CKD-related mineral and bone disorder (CKD-MBD) leads to complex disturbances in calcium, phosphorus, vitamin D, and PTH metabolism, causing renal osteodystrophy and increasing the risk of fragility fractures.

Hematological Disorders

- Conditions like multiple myeloma, leukemia, and lymphoma disrupt bone remodeling directly and through treatment regimens, contributing to severe secondary osteoporosis.

Neurological Disorders and Immobilization

- Prolonged immobility from conditions such as stroke, spinal cord injury, Parkinson's disease, or multiple sclerosis leads to disuse osteoporosis. The absence of mechanical loading reduces bone formation, particularly in weight-bearing skeletal regions.

MEDICATIONS THAT INDUCE BONE LOSS

Several commonly used drugs are known to contribute to secondary osteoporosis:

- **Glucocorticoids**: The most common cause of drug-induced osteoporosis. They reduce osteoblast function, increase osteoclast survival, and impair calcium absorption.
- **Anticonvulsants**: Especially phenytoin and phenobarbital, which increase vitamin D metabolism and reduce its availability.
- **Aromatase inhibitors**: Used in breast cancer treatment, they reduce estrogen levels and accelerate bone loss.
- **Androgen deprivation therapy**: In prostate cancer management, it lowers testosterone levels and compromises bone health.
- **Proton Pump Inhibitors (PPIs)**: Long-term use may impair calcium absorption by reducing gastric acidity.
- **SSRIs**: Selective serotonin reuptake inhibitors have been associated with

lower bone density and increased fracture risk, especially in older adults.

SPECIAL POPULATIONS AT RISK

1. Postmenopausal Women
   - Estrogen plays a central role in bone remodeling. Its sudden withdrawal post-menopause leads to an immediate increase in bone resorption and gradual loss of bone mass, placing women at high risk for osteoporosis and fractures, especially vertebral fractures.

2. Older Adults
   - Elderly individuals often have compounded risk factors: decreased renal function, malabsorption, polypharmacy, frailty, and increased risk of falls. Hip fractures in this group are particularly devastating, often leading to loss of independence and increased mortality.

3. Young Adults and Adolescents
Although less common, osteoporosis can develop in younger individuals due to:
   - Genetic disorders (e.g., osteogenesis imperfecta)

- Eating disorders (e.g., anorexia nervosa)
- Amenorrhea due to athletic or nutritional causes
- Use of corticosteroids or other medications
- Early detection and lifestyle interventions are critical to minimize long-term damage.

Risk Assessment Tools: Several tools help clinicians assess osteoporosis risk and guide decisions about screening and treatment:

FRAX (Fracture Risk Assessment Tool)

- Developed by the WHO, FRAX estimates a 10-year probability of hip and major osteoporotic fractures using clinical risk factors with or without BMD data. It includes age, sex, BMI, smoking status, alcohol use, previous fractures, parental hip fracture history, glucocorticoid use, rheumatoid arthritis, and secondary osteoporosis.

Garvan Fracture Risk Calculator

- This tool provides a 5- and 10-year fracture risk, incorporating similar clinical risk factors along with fall history.

Osteoporosis is a multifactorial disease shaped by a combination of genetic, hormonal, nutritional, lifestyle, and medical factors. While some risks, such as age and sex, are immutable, many others—particularly nutritional deficiencies, physical inactivity, and smoking—are modifiable through education and preventive measures.

Secondary causes of osteoporosis, often overlooked, can significantly contribute to bone loss and must be investigated, especially in younger patients or those with atypical fracture patterns. Clinicians must be vigilant in identifying at-risk individuals and tailoring interventions accordingly. A comprehensive understanding of osteoporosis risk factors equips healthcare providers to implement early prevention strategies, optimize patient outcomes, and reduce the societal burden of this silent epidemic.

CHAPTER 3

CLINICAL PRESENTATION AND COMPLICATIONS

Osteoporosis is often silent until it manifests dramatically through fractures or disabling symptoms. Its insidious nature leads many patients to remain undiagnosed until significant skeletal damage has occurred. Understanding the clinical presentation and recognizing the complications of osteoporosis is crucial for timely diagnosis, appropriate intervention, and prevention of long-term disability. This chapter explores the wide spectrum of clinical features, diagnostic clues, and the complications associated with osteoporosis, ranging from subtle symptoms to life-altering fractures.

THE SILENT NATURE OF OSTEOPOROSIS

Osteoporosis is commonly referred to as a "silent disease" because it progresses asymptomatically until a fragility fracture occurs. Bone loss itself does not cause pain or obvious symptoms. As a result, patients often remain unaware of their condition until irreversible damage has taken place. This characteristic makes early detection challenging and highlights the importance of recognizing early warning signs and risk factors.

CLINICAL PRESENTATION

1. Asymptomatic Phase
In its early stages, osteoporosis does not produce symptoms. During this silent phase:
- Bone mineral density (BMD) gradually declines.
- There is no pain, swelling, or functional limitation.

- Many cases are incidentally discovered during routine imaging or after a fracture.
- Routine screening in at-risk individuals—such as postmenopausal women and older adults—is vital to identifying osteoporosis before complications arise

2. Pain and Postural Changes

Although osteoporosis itself is painless, structural changes in the spine can lead to:

- Back pain: Typically in the thoracic or lumbar regions. This can occur acutely with vertebral fractures or chronically due to postural strain.
- Kyphosis: Commonly known as a "dowager's hump," kyphosis results from multiple anterior vertebral compression fractures. The forward curvature of the upper spine impairs posture and contributes to imbalance.
- Loss of height: Progressive vertebral compression leads to loss of up to several inches in height. Patients often report that clothing no longer fits properly or that they appear shorter in photographs.

- These subtle indicators may precede a diagnosis and should prompt further evaluation in high-risk individuals.

FRAGILITY FRACTURES

The hallmark of clinical osteoporosis is the fragility fracture—a break that occurs from a fall from standing height or less. These fractures commonly occur in the:

a. Vertebrae (Spine)
- Most common site of osteoporotic fractures.
- Often occur silently, with only one-third of patients aware they have sustained a spinal fracture.
- Symptoms include sudden onset of back pain, reduced mobility, difficulty standing upright, and visible spinal deformity.

b. Hip
- One of the most devastating and costly fractures.
- Usually results from a fall in elderly patients with reduced bone density and poor balance.

- Symptoms include severe groin or thigh pain, inability to bear weight, and external rotation of the leg.
- Hip fractures often require surgical intervention and are associated with significant mortality and long-term disability.

c. Wrist (Distal Radius)

- Common in younger postmenopausal women.
- Typically occurs when trying to break a fall with an outstretched hand.
- Leads to pain, swelling, and functional impairment of the hand and wrist.

d. Proximal Humerus and Pelvis

- These sites also represent frequent fragility fractures, particularly in older adults.
- They may result in substantial loss of function and prolonged rehabilitation.

REDUCED MOBILITY AND FUNCTIONAL DECLINE

Following a fracture, patients may experience:
- Prolonged immobility.

- Reduced ability to perform activities of daily living (ADLs).
- Loss of independence, often necessitating assisted living or long-term care placement.
- Deconditioning and sarcopenia (loss of muscle mass), which further compound fall risk and impair recovery.

- The psychological toll of these limitations can be profound and must not be underestimated.

Psychological Impact

Osteoporosis can have significant emotional and psychological effects, including:

- **Fear of falling**: Resulting in reduced activity levels and social withdrawal.
- **Depression**: Due to chronic pain, disability, or loss of independence.
- **Anxiety**: Over the possibility of future fractures or worsening deformity.
- These psychological consequences can severely affect quality of life and should be addressed alongside physical treatment.

COMPLICATIONS OF OSTEOPOROSIS

The complications of osteoporosis can be broadly divided into physical, functional, and psychosocial domains. Many of these complications stem from fragility fractures and can be life-altering.

1. Vertebral Compression Fractures (VCFs): Vertebral fractures are the most common osteoporotic fractures, often occurring without trauma.

a. Pathophysiology

- The vertebral body collapses due to weakened trabecular bone.
- This may happen suddenly or gradually over time.

b. Clinical Features

- Acute or chronic back pain.
- Spinal deformity and kyphosis.
- Loss of height.
- Reduced pulmonary function in severe kyphosis due to restricted lung expansion.

c. Impact

- Even a single VCF increases the risk of subsequent vertebral and non-vertebral fractures.

- Chronic pain and reduced mobility lead to further deconditioning and fracture risk.

2. Hip Fractures

Hip fractures represent a medical emergency in elderly patients and are associated with severe outcomes:

a. Clinical Course

- Requires surgical repair in most cases.
- Frequently followed by prolonged hospitalization and rehabilitation.
- High risk of post-operative complications (e.g., infections, thromboembolism).

b. Outcomes

- Mortality rate of up to 20–30% within one year.
- Less than half of patients regain previous functional status.
- Many require permanent institutional care.

3. Non-Vertebral, Non-Hip Fractures

These include fractures of the:

- Wrist
- Humerus
- Pelvis
- Ribs

While these are less life-threatening, they can still cause considerable morbidity:

- Impaired upper limb function.
- Chronic pain and disability.
- Increased future fracture risk.

4. Chronic Pain Syndrome

Chronic pain following osteoporotic fractures—especially vertebral fractures—can lead to:

- Muscle spasms.
- Sleep disturbances.
- Opioid dependence.
- Psychosocial distress and reduced quality of life.
- Pain management becomes a complex component of osteoporosis care in these patients.

5. Postural Instability and Falls

Fractures lead to muscular atrophy, altered gait, and poor balance. These factors:

- Increase fall risk.
- Perpetuate a cycle of falls and fractures.
- Often necessitate assistive devices and fall-prevention programs.

6. Pulmonary Complications

In severe kyphosis caused by multiple vertebral fractures:

- Lung expansion may be restricted.
- Patients may experience dyspnea on exertion.
- Increased susceptibility to respiratory infections such as pneumonia.

7. Gastrointestinal and Abdominal Issues

Kyphosis can compress abdominal organs, leading to:

- Early satiety and reduced appetite.
- Constipation.
- Gastroesophageal reflux disease (GERD).
- These effects can further impair nutritional status and bone health.

8. Increased Mortality

Numerous studies have linked osteoporosis-related fractures—particularly hip and vertebral fractures—to increased mortality.

Hip Fracture Mortality

- Highest during the first 6 months post-fracture.
- Attributable to immobility, complications, and pre-existing frailty.

Vertebral Fracture Mortality
- Associated with pulmonary dysfunction, immobility, and systemic complications.
- Predicts future fracture risk and mortality.

9. Recurrent Fractures

After an initial osteoporotic fracture:

- The risk of future fractures doubles or triples.
- Approximately 20% of women who sustain a vertebral fracture will have another within the next year.
- The highest risk period is within the first 12–24 months post-fracture.
- This underscores the urgency of initiating treatment after the first fracture.

ATYPICAL PRESENTATIONS AND SPECIAL CONSIDERATIONS

1. Atypical Femur Fractures (AFFs)

Though rare, long-term use of bisphosphonates (antiresorptive therapy) can lead to atypical femoral fractures:

- Often subtrochanteric or femoral shaft fractures.
- Preceded by thigh pain.

- Occur with minimal or no trauma.
- Typically transverse and non-comminuted on imaging.
- Early recognition and drug holiday strategies are important for prevention.

2. Osteonecrosis of the Jaw (ONJ)

Another rare complication linked to antiresorptive therapy:

- More common with intravenous bisphosphonates or denosumab.
- Often follows dental surgery or trauma.
- Presents with jaw pain, exposed bone, and non-healing lesions.
- Preventive dental evaluation and hygiene are recommended before starting high-potency osteoporosis treatments.

3. Comorbidities Impacting Presentation

Patients with comorbid conditions (e.g., rheumatoid arthritis, chronic kidney disease, Parkinson's disease) may present with compounded symptoms:

- Greater fall risk.
- Drug interactions.
- Overlapping musculoskeletal symptoms, masking osteoporosis.

- These patients require multidisciplinary evaluation and tailored treatment strategies.

DIAGNOSTIC CLUES AND EVALUATION AFTER PRESENTATION

Once osteoporosis is suspected or a fragility fracture is identified, further evaluation is warranted:

a. Bone Mineral Density Testing

- Dual-energy X-ray absorptiometry (DXA) is the gold standard.
- Measures BMD at the hip and spine.
- T-score ≤ -2.5 confirms osteoporosis.

b. Spinal Imaging

- X-rays to assess for vertebral compression fractures.
- Vertebral fracture assessment (VFA) during DXA scans.

c. Laboratory Tests

- Serum calcium, phosphate, 25(OH) vitamin D.
- PTH, thyroid function, renal and liver panels.

- Consider secondary causes if fractures are atypical or occur in young patients.

Osteoporosis, though initially silent, eventually presents with serious and often life-altering complications. Fragility fractures—especially of the spine and hip—are the primary clinical manifestations and serve as crucial signals for intervention. Chronic pain, physical disability, loss of independence, and even death are common consequences of advanced disease.

Clinicians must be vigilant in recognizing early warning signs, screening at-risk populations, and addressing complications promptly and holistically. Beyond pharmacologic therapy, management requires a comprehensive approach that includes pain control, rehabilitation, psychological support, and fall prevention to restore function and preserve quality of life.

CHAPTER 4

DIAGNOSIS AND SCREENING

Osteoporosis often progresses silently until a fracture occurs, making early diagnosis and screening critical for effective management and prevention of complications. This chapter delves into the diagnostic strategies and screening guidelines that help identify osteoporosis early, thus allowing timely intervention. We will explore the tools, technologies, clinical assessments, and evolving best practices used to detect low bone density and assess fracture risk.

IMPORTANCE OF EARLY DIAGNOSIS

Osteoporosis is frequently termed a "silent disease" because bone loss occurs without symptoms. By the time fractures occur, the disease is often already advanced. Early diagnosis enables:

- Initiation of lifestyle changes or pharmacologic treatments
- Prevention of fractures and their associated morbidity
- Monitoring of treatment efficacy and disease progression
- Early identification is particularly vital in populations at increased risk such as postmenopausal women, older adults, and individuals with secondary causes of osteoporosis.

CLINICAL EVALUATION AND RISK ASSESSMENT

The first step in diagnosing osteoporosis involves a detailed medical history and physical examination. Clinicians should assess for:

A. Risk Factors

- **Age and sex**: Women over 65 and men over 70 are at increased risk.
- **Family history**: Especially parental history of hip fractures.
- **Lifestyle factors**: Low body weight, smoking, alcohol use, physical inactivity.
- **Medical history**: Early menopause, glucocorticoid use, rheumatoid arthritis, gastrointestinal disorders affecting absorption.
- **Fracture history**: Prior fragility fracture is a strong predictor of future fractures.

B. Physical Examination

Though limited in diagnosing osteoporosis directly, physical examination can uncover indicators such as:

- Height loss >2 cm
- Kyphosis or dowager's hump
- Balance issues increasing fall risk
- A complete evaluation sets the stage for targeted diagnostic testing.

BONE MINERAL DENSITY TESTING

The cornerstone of osteoporosis diagnosis is bone mineral density (BMD) testing, typically using dual-energy X-ray absorptiometry (DXA or DEXA).

A. Dual-Energy X-ray Absorptiometry (DXA)

- Gold standard test for measuring BMD.
- Typically assesses the lumbar spine, total hip, and femoral neck.
- T-score and Z-score values are derived from BMD results.

- T-score interpretation (for postmenopausal women and men ≥50 years)
- Normal: T-score ≥ -1.0
- Osteopenia (low bone mass): T-score between -1.0 and -2.5
- Osteoporosis: T-score ≤ -2.5
- Severe osteoporosis: T-score ≤ -2.5 with a fragility fracture
- Z-score interpretation (for premenopausal women and men <50 years)

- Compares BMD to age- and sex-matched norms.
- Z-score < -2.0 may suggest secondary osteoporosis.
- DXA is safe, quick, and uses minimal radiation.

B. Peripheral DXA (pDXA) and Quantitative Ultrasound

- pDXA measures BMD at peripheral sites (e.g., forearm, heel).
- Quantitative ultrasound (QUS) assesses bone properties in the heel using sound waves.
- These are useful for screening in settings without access to central DXA but are not diagnostic substitutes.

Vertebral Fracture Assessment (VFA)

As many vertebral fractures are asymptomatic, vertebral fracture assessment (VFA) using DXA imaging of the spine is a valuable tool. VFA can be performed simultaneously with BMD testing.

- Useful in identifying previously undiagnosed fractures.
- Indicated in patients with height loss, kyphosis, or low BMD.

- Detects fractures that may change management, even if T-score > -2.5.

Biochemical Markers of Bone Turnover
Though not diagnostic, biochemical markers are increasingly used to assess bone metabolism and monitor therapy response.
- Bone Formation Markers
- Serum osteocalcin
- Bone-specific alkaline phosphatase (BSAP)
- Procollagen type 1 N-terminal propeptide (P1NP)

- Bone Resorption Markers
- Urinary or serum C-terminal telopeptide (CTX)
- N-terminal telopeptide (NTX)
- While these markers exhibit variability, they provide insight into bone turnover dynamics, particularly in therapy monitoring.

SCREENING GUIDELINES AND RECOMMENDATIONS

Screening is aimed at identifying individuals at risk before clinical manifestations occur. Recommendations vary slightly between organizations but share common principles.

A. U.S. Preventive Services Task Force (USPSTF)

- Women ≥65 years: Routine BMD screening.
- Younger women (50–64): If fracture risk is equal to or greater than that of a 65-year-old woman.
- Insufficient evidence for routine screening in men, but clinical judgment is advised.

B. National Osteoporosis Foundation (NOF)

- Women ≥65 and men ≥70
- Postmenopausal women and men 50–69 with risk factors
- Adults with a fracture after age 50
- Adults with conditions or medications associated with bone loss

Screening intervals may vary:
- Every 2 years is typical, but shorter intervals may apply in high-risk patients or to monitor treatment.

Fracture Risk Assessment Tools
- To supplement BMD data, tools such as FRAX estimate 10-year probability of fracture.
- FRAX (Fracture Risk Assessment Tool)
- Developed by the WHO.
- Integrates clinical risk factors with or without BMD.
- Outputs 10-year probability of:
- Hip fracture
- Major osteoporotic fracture (hip, spine, forearm, or shoulder)

Key Inputs
- Age, sex, BMI
- Prior fractures
- Parental hip fracture
- Smoking
- Glucocorticoid use
- Rheumatoid arthritis

- Alcohol intake
- Secondary osteoporosis
- Femoral neck BMD (optional but improves accuracy)
- Thresholds for Intervention
- Major osteoporotic fracture risk ≥20% or hip fracture risk ≥3% generally warrants treatment.
- FRAX aids clinicians in decision-making, especially when BMD alone is borderline.

EMERGING AND ADJUNIVE DIAGNOSTIC TOOLS

A. Trabecular Bone Score (TBS)
- Derived from DXA images of the lumbar spine.
- Provides information about bone microarchitecture, independent of BMD.
- Lower TBS indicates degraded bone quality and higher fracture risk.

Useful in:
- Older adults
- Diabetics
- Patients on corticosteroids

B. Quantitative Computed Tomography (QCT)

- Measures volumetric BMD.
- Better at assessing trabecular bone and differentiating between cortical and trabecular loss.
- Used mostly in research or complex clinical cases.

C. High-Resolution Peripheral QCT (HR-pQCT)

- Provides microstructural bone details.
- Limited to research settings, but holds promise for future diagnostics.

Diagnosing Secondary Osteoporosis

In cases where osteoporosis is suspected due to secondary causes (especially in younger patients or men), a thorough laboratory workup is necessary to identify underlying conditions. Common Tests

- Calcium, phosphate, and vitamin D levels
- Parathyroid hormone (PTH)
- Thyroid-stimulating hormone (TSH)
- Serum protein electrophoresis (SPEP) for multiple myeloma

- Liver and kidney function tests
- Testosterone and estradiol levels
- Uncovering secondary causes is crucial because treating the underlying disorder may halt or reverse bone loss.

CHALLENGES IN SCREENING AND DIAGNOSIS

Despite available tools, osteoporosis often goes undiagnosed due to:
- Lack of symptoms until fracture
- Underutilization of DXA testing
- Limited awareness among men and younger at-risk populations
- Geographical and economic barriers to access
- Healthcare systems must work to improve public awareness, facilitate access to screening, and prioritize at-risk individuals.

Strategies for Improving Early Identification
To overcome diagnostic delays, the following strategies are recommended:
- Fracture Liaison Services (FLS): Coordinated post-fracture care to assess BMD and initiate treatment.

- Opportunistic screening: Use spine imaging or chest X-rays to identify vertebral fractures.
- Electronic medical record alerts: Automated reminders for screening in eligible patients.
- Public health campaigns: Encourage screening especially among older adults.
- Early diagnosis through these means can substantially reduce fracture risk and improve long-term outcomes.

Osteoporosis can remain undetected for years until significant, life-altering fractures occur. Therefore, timely diagnosis and screening are essential components of osteoporosis management. Tools such as DXA, FRAX, and laboratory evaluations provide a comprehensive view of an individual's bone health and fracture risk. With increased awareness, utilization of screening guidelines, and integration of emerging technologies, healthcare providers can identify osteoporosis earlier, initiate appropriate interventions, and prevent debilitating complications. In the evolving landscape of bone health, prioritizing early detection remains the cornerstone of effective osteoporosis care.

CHAPTER 5

LIFESTYLE MODIFICATIONS

While pharmacologic therapies play a crucial role in osteoporosis treatment, lifestyle modifications form the foundation of comprehensive management. These non-pharmacologic strategies are critical not only for preventing bone loss but also for enhancing overall musculoskeletal health, improving quality of life, and reducing the risk of falls and fractures. In this chapter, we explore the key elements of lifestyle modification—including nutrition, physical activity, smoking cessation, alcohol moderation, fall prevention, and other behavioral interventions—that support bone health and complement clinical treatments.

IMPORTANCE OF LIFESTYLE MODIFICATIONS

Lifestyle changes are essential because:
- Bone health is dynamic and influenced by everyday habits.

- Medications are more effective when supported by proper diet and exercise.
- Prevention is more cost-effective and less invasive than treating fractures.
- Lifelong habits formed early help prevent osteoporosis later in life.

Thus, lifestyle interventions should be individualized and implemented early, ideally beginning in childhood and continuing through adulthood.

NUTRITIONAL OPTIMIZATION

A. Calcium Intake

- Calcium is the primary mineral in bone, making it vital for maintaining bone mass.
- Recommended Daily Intake
- Adults aged 19–50: 1,000 mg/day
- Women ≥51 and men ≥71: 1,200 mg/day

Dietary Sources

- Dairy: milk, yogurt, cheese
- Leafy greens: kale, collard greens
- Fortified foods: juices, cereals, plant-based milk
- Fish with bones: sardines, salmon

- If dietary intake is insufficient, supplements may be used, preferably divided into two doses of 500–600 mg each to enhance absorption. Calcium carbonate (taken with food) and calcium citrate (better absorbed without food) are common options.

B. Vitamin D

Vitamin D facilitates calcium absorption in the intestines and is vital for bone remodeling.
Recommended Intake

- Adults ≤70: 600 IU/day
- Adults >70: 800 IU/day

Sources

- Sunlight exposure (10–30 minutes/day, depending on skin tone and geography)
- Fatty fish, egg yolks, fortified foods
- Supplements: vitamin D2 or D3 (D3 is preferred)
- Vitamin D deficiency is common, particularly in the elderly or those with limited sun exposure. Serum 25-hydroxyvitamin D levels should ideally be >30 ng/mL. Supplementation may range from 1,000–2,000 IU/day, or higher for

deficient individuals under medical supervision.

C. Other Nutrients

Protein

- Adequate intake (1.0–1.2 g/kg/day) supports muscle strength and bone health.
- Both animal and plant sources are beneficial when calcium intake is sufficient.
- Magnesium, Potassium, and Phosphorus
- Found in whole grains, nuts, fruits, and vegetables.
- Support bone metabolism and density.

Vitamin K

- Important in osteocalcin regulation, a protein critical for bone formation.
- Found in green leafy vegetables.
- Balanced, nutrient-dense diets such as the Mediterranean diet offer protective effects against osteoporosis.

PHYSICAL ACTIVITY AND EXERCISE

A. Benefits of Exercise

- Regular physical activity:

- Stimulates bone formation
- Increases muscle strength
- Enhances balance and coordination
- Reduces risk of falls and fractures

B. Types of Recommended Exercises

- Weight-Bearing Exercises
- Activities that make you move against gravity while upright
- Examples: brisk walking, hiking, dancing, stair climbing
- Recommended: 30 minutes/day, 5 days/week
- Resistance (Strength) Training
- Builds muscle mass and strengthens bones
- Uses weights, resistance bands, or body weight
- Targets spine, hips, and wrists—common fracture sites
- Recommended: 2–3 times/week
- Balance and Flexibility Training
- Improves proprioception and reduces fall risk
- Includes yoga, tai chi, Pilates
- Especially valuable in the elderly

Postural Training

- Aids in preventing kyphosis and vertebral fractures
- Encourages spine-stabilizing activities like wall sits or posture drills
- Exercise regimens should be tailored to individual capacity, avoiding high-impact or twisting movements in those with severe osteoporosis.

SMOKING CESSATION

A. Effects of Smoking on Bone Health
- Smoking reduces estrogen levels in women, impairing bone formation.
- It affects osteoblast activity, reducing new bone formation.
- Increases production of cortisol, which promotes bone resorption.
- Decreases calcium absorption and reduces vitamin D metabolism.
- Smokers are at significantly higher risk of fractures and poorer healing outcomes. Quitting smoking has been shown to improve BMD over time and should be a key component of osteoporosis management.

Alcohol Moderation

Excessive alcohol intake negatively impacts bone health by:

- Inhibiting osteoblast function
- Increasing risk of falls due to impaired coordination
- Affecting calcium metabolism and vitamin D levels

Recommended Limits

- Women: ≤1 drink/day

- Men: ≤2 drinks/day

- Patients with osteoporosis should be counseled on the impact of alcohol and encouraged to drink in moderation or abstain if necessary.

FALL PREVENTION STRATEGIES

Falls are the leading cause of fractures in people with osteoporosis. Preventing falls is therefore a key goal of lifestyle modification.

A. Home Safety Modifications

- Remove clutter, loose rugs, and electrical cords
- Install grab bars in bathrooms and handrails on stairs

- Ensure proper lighting throughout the home
- Use nonslip mats in bathtubs and kitchens

B. Assistive Devices

- Canes, walkers, and supportive footwear help reduce fall risk
- Medical alert systems can provide emergency support

C. Vision and Hearing

- Regular eye exams and hearing checks reduce sensory-related fall risk

D. Medication Review

- Sedatives, antihypertensives, and certain psychotropic drugs may increase fall risk
- Regular medication reviews help minimize side effects

E. Balance Training

- Tai chi and other balance-focused exercises enhance neuromuscular coordination
- Fall prevention efforts must be personalized and reassessed regularly as patients age or their health status changes.

BODY WEIGHT AND COMPOSITION
A. Low Body Weight

- BMI <20 is associated with reduced BMD and increased fracture risk
- Adequate caloric intake is essential for bone formation

B. Obesity
- While excess weight may protect against osteoporosis in some sites, it increases risk of falls and mobility issues
- Central obesity may promote inflammation that contributes to bone loss
- A balanced approach to weight management—avoiding extremes—is ideal for bone health.

Caffeine and Soda Consumption
A. Caffeine
- High caffeine intake may modestly reduce calcium absorption
- Limit to <3 cups of coffee/day, especially if calcium intake is low

B. Carbonated Beverages

- Excessive consumption of colas, especially those with phosphoric acid, may negatively affect bone

- Encourage milk, water, or calcium-fortified alternatives instead
- Education about these dietary choices is important, especially in adolescents and young adults forming bone mass.

SUNLIGHT AND OUTDOOR ACTIVITY

Regular sunlight exposure promotes endogenous vitamin D synthesis, which is critical for calcium absorption.

- Aim for 10–30 minutes of sun exposure on face and arms 3–5 times per week
- Caution must be balanced with skin cancer prevention in fair-skinned individuals
- Outdoor activities also increase physical activity and improve mood
- For those with limited sun exposure, vitamin D supplementation is essential.

Psychological Wellbeing and Motivation

Osteoporosis can be associated with depression, fear of falling, and social withdrawal. Addressing mental health is vital in comprehensive care.

A. Counseling and Support Groups

- Help patients cope with chronic illness
- Improve adherence to lifestyle recommendations

B. Education

- Increases understanding of disease and empowers self-management
- Patients educated on risk factors are more likely to adopt lifestyle changes

INTEGRATING LIFESTYLE CHANGES INTO DAILY LIFE

The key to successful lifestyle modification is sustainability and personalization.

A. Goal-Setting and Monitoring

- Establish realistic, incremental goals
- Use apps, journals, or wearable devices to track progress

B. Multidisciplinary Support

- Dietitians, physiotherapists, occupational therapists, and health coaches can reinforce behavior change

C. Family and Community Involvement

- Involving family helps reinforce positive habits
- Community programs (e.g., fall prevention classes, walking groups) increase adherence
- Lifestyle change is a lifelong journey that evolves with age, health status, and treatment goals.

Lifestyle modification is not merely an adjunct but a cornerstone of osteoporosis management. Nutrition, exercise, fall prevention, and behavioral changes provide foundational support for both prevention and treatment. These interventions are cost-effective, low-risk, and highly beneficial across all age groups. By empowering individuals to make informed choices and sustain healthy habits, clinicians can help reduce fracture incidence, preserve independence, and improve overall quality of life. A commitment to lifestyle modification, reinforced by ongoing support and education, is essential in the fight against osteoporosis.

CHAPTER 6

PHARMACOLOGIC THERAPY

Osteoporosis is a chronic condition marked by reduced bone mineral density and structural deterioration of bone tissue, leading to increased bone fragility and risk of fractures. While lifestyle interventions are foundational, many individuals—particularly those with moderate to severe bone loss or high fracture risk—require pharmacologic therapy to arrest disease progression and reduce fracture risk. This chapter explores the spectrum of medications used in osteoporosis management, including their mechanisms, indications, benefits, limitations, and monitoring protocols.

GOALS OF PHARMACOLOGIC THERAPY

Pharmacologic treatment aims to:

- Prevent fractures, especially vertebral and hip fractures.
- Increase or maintain bone mineral density (BMD).
- Reduce bone resorption or stimulate bone formation.
- Improve quality of life by preventing loss of mobility and independence.
- Treatment choice is guided by the patient's age, sex, fracture history, BMD scores (T-scores), FRAX (Fracture Risk Assessment Tool) results, menopausal status, and comorbidities.

CATEGORIES OF OSTEOPOROSIS MEDICATIONS

Pharmacologic therapies fall into two main categories:

A. Antiresorptive Agents

- These medications slow bone resorption by inhibiting osteoclast activity.
- Bisphosphonates
- Selective Estrogen Receptor Modulators (SERMs)
- Denosumab
- Hormone Replacement Therapy (HRT)

- Calcitonin

B. Anabolic (Bone-Forming) Agents

These drugs stimulate new bone formation by enhancing osteoblast activity.

- Teriparatide
- Abaloparatide
- Romosozumab
- The choice of therapy depends on individual fracture risk, tolerance, cost, and medical contraindications.

BISPHOSPHONATES

A. Mechanism of Action

- Bisphosphonates bind to bone mineral surfaces and inhibit osteoclast-mediated bone resorption, preserving bone mass and improving BMD.

B. Common Bisphosphonates

- Alendronate (oral, weekly)
- Risedronate (oral, weekly or monthly)
- Ibandronate (oral monthly or IV quarterly)
- Zoledronic acid (IV yearly)

C. Indications

- Postmenopausal women and men with osteoporosis
- Individuals with prior fragility fractures

- Glucocorticoid-induced osteoporosis

D. Benefits
- Reduce vertebral fractures by 40–70%
- Reduce hip fractures by 20–50%
- Long half-life allows for infrequent dosing

E. Side Effects and Risks
- Gastrointestinal irritation (oral forms)
- Acute phase reactions (IV forms)
- Rare but serious: osteonecrosis of the jaw (ONJ) and atypical femoral fractures (with long-term use)

F. Considerations
- Administer oral agents with water on an empty stomach, remain upright for 30–60 minutes.
- Drug holidays may be considered after 3–5 years in low-risk patients.

DENOSUMAB

A. Mechanism of Action
- A monoclonal antibody that inhibits RANKL, a key protein in osteoclast activation, thus preventing bone resorption.

B. Brand Name

- Prolia (60 mg subcutaneous injection every 6 months)

C. Indications

- Postmenopausal women at high risk of fracture
- Men with osteoporosis
- Individuals intolerant to bisphosphonates

D. Benefits

- Reduces vertebral, non-vertebral, and hip fractures
- Does not accumulate in bone, allowing for rapid reversibility

E. Side Effects and Risks

- Hypocalcemia (especially in renal impairment)
- Increased risk of infection
- ONJ and atypical fractures (similar to bisphosphonates)
- Rebound vertebral fractures if therapy is stopped abruptly

F. Monitoring

- Ensure adequate calcium and vitamin D intake
- Monitor serum calcium and renal function before injection

Selective Estrogen Receptor Modulators (SERMs)

A. Mechanism of Action

- SERMs mimic estrogen's positive effects on bone while avoiding its risks to breast and uterine tissue.

B. Common SERM

- Raloxifene (60 mg oral daily)

C. Indications

- Postmenopausal women with vertebral fracture risk
- Women who cannot tolerate other therapies

D. Benefits

- Reduces vertebral fractures by ~30%
- No stimulation of endometrium or breast tissue
- May reduce breast cancer risk

E. Risks and Side Effects

- Hot flashes, leg cramps
- Increased risk of venous thromboembolism
- Does not reduce hip fracture risk

HORMONE REPLACEMENT THERAPY (HRT)

A. Mechanism of Action

- Estrogen reduces bone resorption and maintains BMD in postmenopausal women.

B. Indications

- Women with menopausal symptoms and high fracture risk
- Short-term use in early menopause (generally <60 years of age)

C. Benefits

- Improves BMD
- Relieves menopausal symptoms

D. Risks

- Increased risk of breast cancer, stroke, heart disease, and venous thromboembolism
- Requires individual risk-benefit assessment

CALCITONIN

A. Mechanism of Action

- A hormone that directly inhibits osteoclast activity.

B. Formulation
- Nasal spray (200 IU daily) or subcutaneous injection

C. Indications
- Women >5 years post-menopause with osteoporosis
- Short-term use for acute pain from vertebral fractures

D. Benefits and Limitations
- Modest efficacy in reducing vertebral fractures
- No proven benefit for hip fractures
- Less commonly used due to weak effect and cancer risk concerns

Anabolic Therapies

These therapies are reserved for individuals with severe osteoporosis, multiple fractures, or failure of antiresorptive agents.

A. Teriparatide
- Mechanism
- Recombinant PTH (parathyroid hormone)
- Stimulates osteoblasts to build new bone
- Dose and Administration
- 20 mcg daily subcutaneous injection for up to 2 years

Indications

- Severe osteoporosis with high fracture risk
- Glucocorticoid-induced osteoporosis

Benefits

- Reduces vertebral fractures by 65% and nonvertebral by 53%
- Increases BMD substantially

Risks

- Hypercalcemia
- Leg cramps, nausea
- Theoretical risk of osteosarcoma (seen in rats, not confirmed in humans)

B. Abaloparatide

Mechanism

- Analog of PTHrP (parathyroid hormone-related protein)
- Similar action to teriparatide

Administration

- 80 mcg daily subcutaneous injection

Benefits and Risks

- Comparable to teriparatide in fracture reduction
- May cause hypercalciuria and dizziness

C. Romosozumab

Mechanism

- Monoclonal antibody that inhibits sclerostin, enhancing bone formation and reducing resorption

Dose
- 210 mg subcutaneous monthly for 12 months

Indications
- Postmenopausal women with high fracture risk

Benefits
- Greater BMD increases than other agents
- Reduces vertebral fracture risk by up to 73%

Risks
- Potential increased cardiovascular risk (stroke, MI)
- Reserved for patients without recent heart events

SEQUENTIAL AND COMBINATION THERAPY

Due to different mechanisms, medications may be used sequentially or in combination:

A. Sequential Therapy

- Start with anabolic (e.g., teriparatide) → follow with antiresorptive (e.g., bisphosphonate) to maintain gains

B. Combination Therapy

- Limited benefit and increased cost
- Used in rare cases of extremely high fracture risk

C. Transition Considerations

- Discontinuing denosumab abruptly can cause rapid bone loss
- Transition to bisphosphonates helps retain BMD

Monitoring and Adherence

A. Monitoring

- DEXA scan every 1–2 years to assess BMD response
- FRAX reassessment to adjust treatment intensity
- Monitor calcium, vitamin D, renal function, and markers of bone turnover as needed

B. Adherence Challenges

- Oral bisphosphonates have complex dosing
- Injections require scheduling
- Side effects may reduce compliance

C. Solutions
- Education on fracture risk reduction
- Simplify regimens where possible
- Address concerns about long-term effects

SPECIAL POPULATIONS

A. Men with Osteoporosis
- Often underdiagnosed
- Treat with bisphosphonates, denosumab, or teriparatide

B. Glucocorticoid-Induced Osteoporosis
- Common in chronic steroid users
- Early prevention and treatment critical

C. Chronic Kidney Disease (CKD)
- Some therapies (e.g., bisphosphonates) must be used cautiously or avoided
- Denosumab or anabolic agents may be preferred in certain CKD stages

Pharmacologic therapy represents a pivotal component of osteoporosis management, especially for individuals with high fracture risk or severe bone loss. A wide range of medications—including antiresorptive and anabolic agents—are available, allowing personalized and evidence-based treatment plans. With proper selection, monitoring, and adherence support, these therapies significantly reduce the risk of fractures and preserve quality of life. However, medication use must always be integrated with lifestyle changes and regular follow-up to maximize effectiveness and minimize adverse outcomes.

CHAPTER 7

MANAGEMENT OF OSTEOPOROSIS FRACTURES

Osteoporosis, characterized by diminished bone density and structural deterioration, often reveals itself not through laboratory findings or imaging alone but through its most devastating consequence—fractures. Osteoporotic fractures, particularly of the hip, vertebrae, and wrist, impose immense burdens on individuals, families, and healthcare systems. Managing these fractures requires a multidimensional approach encompassing acute care, rehabilitation, secondary prevention, and often long-term lifestyle adjustments.

In this chapter, we explore in detail the types of osteoporotic fractures, their clinical implications, acute and chronic management strategies, and approaches for preventing future fractures.

THE BURDEN OF OSTEOPOROSIS FRACTURES

1. The Burden of Osteoporotic Fractures
Epidemiological Impact

- Over 8.9 million fractures worldwide are attributed to osteoporosis each year.
- One in three women and one in five men over age 50 will experience an osteoporotic fracture in their lifetime.
- Hip fractures, though less common than vertebral fractures, are more lethal, with a one-year mortality of 20–30%.

Common Sites

- Vertebral Compression Fractures (VCFs)
- Hip Fractures (femoral neck and intertrochanteric)
- Wrist Fractures (distal radius)
- Humerus, pelvis, and ribs
- Each location demands a tailored management strategy based on

functional impact, healing time, and associated complications.

Vertebral Compression Fractures (VCFs)
A. Presentation
- Sudden onset back pain after minimal trauma or none at all
- Height loss, kyphosis ("dowager's hump")
- Functional impairment, reduced pulmonary function in severe cases

B. Diagnosis
- Spinal X-ray or MRI to assess for edema, compression degree
- Bone density testing to confirm osteoporosis

C. Management
Conservative Treatment
- Pain control: NSAIDs, acetaminophen, short-term opioids
- Bracing: Thoracolumbosacral orthosis (TLSO) may offer temporary support
- Physical therapy: Emphasis on postural training, gentle spinal extension exercises

Pharmacologic Therapy

- Calcitonin may be used short-term for analgesia
- Long-term osteoporosis management (bisphosphonates, denosumab, etc.)

Surgical Intervention

Vertebroplasty and kyphoplasty:
- Indicated for persistent pain or functional decline
- Cement injected into fractured vertebra to stabilize and reduce pain
- Controversial efficacy; selection criteria critical

D. Complications
- Chronic pain
- Progressive spinal deformity
- Increased risk of subsequent vertebral fractures

3. Hip Fractures

Presentation
- Inability to bear weight
- Shortened, externally rotated leg
- Pain in groin or hip

Diagnosis
- X-ray confirms fracture location (femoral neck or intertrochanteric)

- MRI or CT if X-ray is inconclusive but suspicion remains high

Management

i. Surgical Treatment

- Femoral Neck Fracture:
- Hemiarthroplasty or total hip replacement (THR)
- Intertrochanteric Fracture:
- Internal fixation with dynamic hip screws or intramedullary nails
- Prompt surgery (within 24–48 hours) reduces mortality and complications.

ii. Postoperative Care

- Early mobilization with physical therapy
- Fall prevention strategies
- DVT prophylaxis
- Pain management

iii. Secondary Prevention

- Start or resume anti-osteoporosis medications post-surgery
- Address nutritional needs (calcium, vitamin D, protein)

D. Complications

- High risk of morbidity and mortality
- Delirium, pressure ulcers, infections
- Long-term loss of independence

4. Wrist and Other Peripheral Fractures
Presentation and Diagnosis
- Distal radius fractures commonly occur from falls on outstretched hands
- Confirmed via X-ray

Treatment
- Closed reduction and casting for stable fractures
- Surgical fixation (e.g., volar plating) for displaced or unstable fractures
- Occupational therapy for regaining hand function

Implications
- Often the first sign of underlying osteoporosis, especially in postmenopausal women
- Should prompt fracture risk assessment and bone density evaluation

ACUTE FRACTURE MANAGEMENT

Regardless of fracture type, initial management principles include:

A. Pain Management
- Acetaminophen, NSAIDs, opioids (short-term only)

- Nerve blocks for hip fractures
- Consider adjuncts like calcitonin for vertebral fractures

B. Mobilization
- Early mobilization reduces risks of DVT, pneumonia, pressure sores
- Geriatric consultation and physical therapy can guide safe transitions

C. Nutritional Support
- Adequate caloric and protein intake promotes healing
- Vitamin D and calcium supplementation essential

D. Psychosocial Considerations
- Many patients experience anxiety, depression, or PTSD post-fracture
- Addressing mental health is key to full recovery

Rehabilitation and Functional Recovery
A. Goals
- Restore baseline function or as close to it as possible
- Prevent future falls and fractures
- Enhance quality of life

B. Physical Therapy

- Strength training, balance exercises, gait training
- Use of assistive devices (walkers, canes) as needed

C. Occupational Therapy
- Focus on activities of daily living (ADLs)
- Home safety evaluations and modifications

D. Multidisciplinary Approach
- Involving physicians, physical therapists, nutritionists, and social workers
- Especially vital for older adults or those with multiple comorbidities

PREVENTING FUTURE FRACTURES (SECONDARY PREVENTION)

A. Initiate or Optimize Osteoporosis Therapy
- Tailor pharmacologic treatment based on risk profile
- Ensure adherence and monitor response

B. Fall Prevention Strategies
- Home safety assessments (remove tripping hazards, improve lighting)
- Vision correction and footwear advice
- Balance and strength training programs (e.g., Tai Chi)

C. Address Modifiable Risk Factors
- Reduce alcohol and tobacco use
- Treat underlying conditions (e.g., Parkinson's, diabetes)
- Review medications that may increase fall risk (sedatives, antihypertensives)

Surgical vs. Non-Surgical Decision-Making
A. Factors Favoring Surgery
- Displaced fractures with instability
- Inability to mobilize conservatively
- Severe pain unresponsive to medical treatment

B. Non-Surgical Indications
- Stable fractures
- Poor surgical candidates (due to comorbidities)
- Patient preference after risk-benefit discussion

The Role of Fracture Liaison Services (FLS)
Fracture Liaison Services provide coordinated post-fracture care aimed at:
- Ensuring BMD testing and osteoporosis treatment initiation
- Monitoring treatment adherence

- Providing fall prevention resources
- FLS programs have demonstrated success in reducing re-fracture rates and improving long-term outcomes.

SPECIAL POPULATIONS

A. The Elderly
- Higher complication rates
- Cognitive impairment may complicate rehabilitation
- Greater need for caregiver support and home adaptations

B. Men with Osteoporotic Fractures
- Often under-recognized and undertreated
- Testosterone levels should be evaluated

C. Patients with Multiple Fractures
- Consider anabolic therapy for enhanced bone healing
- Address frailty and functional decline aggressively

Quality of Life and Psychological Impact
A. Emotional Toll
- Fear of falling again can cause withdrawal and inactivity

- Depression and anxiety are common post-fracture

B. Support Systems
- Counseling and mental health support
- Peer support groups
- Education on osteoporosis and empowerment strategies

The management of osteoporotic fractures demands more than just bone healing—it requires a comprehensive approach that includes acute care, rehabilitation, pharmacologic therapy, fall prevention, and long-term follow-up. Fractures are not only a physical event but a turning point in an individual's trajectory of health and independence. Proactive strategies, multidisciplinary care, and ongoing patient education can dramatically improve outcomes, reduce recurrence, and ultimately, transform a potentially debilitating condition into a manageable one.

CHAPTER 8

SECONDARY OSTEOPOROSIS

Osteoporosis is commonly thought of as a primary disease, particularly affecting postmenopausal women and elderly individuals. However, a substantial proportion of osteoporosis cases—estimated at up to 30–60% in men and 20–40% in women—are attributable to secondary causes. Secondary osteoporosis results from identifiable, often modifiable medical conditions or medications that interfere with bone remodeling or lead to increased bone resorption. Early recognition of these causes is essential to ensure accurate diagnosis, targeted therapy, and fracture prevention.

This chapter will delve into the epidemiology, pathophysiology, diagnostic approach, and management of secondary osteoporosis by examining the key systemic disorders and pharmacologic agents involved.

UNDERSTANDING SECONDARY OSTEOPOROSIS

A. Definition
- Secondary osteoporosis refers to bone loss caused or exacerbated by a specific medical condition, nutritional deficiency, or medication, rather than natural aging or hormonal changes alone.

B. Significance
- Secondary causes are more common in men and younger adults with osteoporosis.
- Failure to identify secondary osteoporosis may result in suboptimal treatment and persistent bone loss.

C. Mechanisms
- Altered bone remodeling (e.g., suppressed osteoblast activity)
- Hormonal imbalances (e.g., excess cortisol, thyroid hormones)

- Nutritional deficiencies (e.g., calcium, vitamin D)
- Direct toxic effects on bone or bone marrow

ENDOCRINE DISORDERS

A. Hyperthyroidism

- Excess thyroid hormones accelerate bone turnover and lead to net bone loss.
- Both overt and subclinical hyperthyroidism are associated with increased fracture risk.
- Treatment: Manage thyroid dysfunction; monitor BMD.

B. Hyperparathyroidism

- In primary hyperparathyroidism, elevated parathyroid hormone (PTH) levels cause cortical bone resorption.
- Patients may present with osteopenia, nephrolithiasis, or vertebral fractures.
- Treatment: Parathyroidectomy or medical management with calcimimetics (e.g., cinacalcet).

C. Cushing's Syndrome

- Endogenous or exogenous glucocorticoid excess leads to suppressed osteoblast activity and increased resorption.
- Osteoporosis is often an early manifestation.
- Treatment: Address the cortisol excess, reduce steroid doses when possible.

D. Hypogonadism

- Estrogen and testosterone are essential for bone health.
- Hypogonadism in men and premenopausal women is a leading cause of secondary osteoporosis.
- Treatment: Hormone replacement therapy if indicated and safe.

E. Diabetes Mellitus

- Type 1 diabetes is associated with low BMD and increased fracture risk.
- Type 2 diabetes often shows normal/high BMD but reduced bone quality.
- Management: Optimize glycemic control, monitor fall risk.

GASTROINTESTINAL AND NUTRITIONAL DISORDERS

A. Malabsorption Syndromes

- Conditions like celiac disease, inflammatory bowel disease (IBD), and chronic pancreatitis impair calcium and vitamin D absorption.
- Chronic inflammation further promotes bone loss.

- Screening: Tissue transglutaminase antibody for celiac disease; colonoscopy for IBD.
- Management: Treat underlying condition, supplement nutrients, and consider antiresorptive therapy.

B. Anorexia Nervosa

- Severe calorie restriction, low BMI, and hypogonadism lead to early-onset osteoporosis.
- Treatment: Nutritional rehabilitation, behavioral therapy, and endocrine support.

C. Vitamin D Deficiency

- Leads to secondary hyperparathyroidism and impaired calcium absorption.
- Particularly common in the elderly, individuals with limited sun exposure, or darker skin tones.

- Diagnosis: Serum 25(OH)D level < 20 ng/mL.
- Treatment: Vitamin D supplementation, typically 800–2000 IU/day.

RENAL AND HEPATIC DISORDERS

A. Chronic Kidney Disease (CKD)
- Associated with complex bone disorders collectively known as renal osteodystrophy.
- Includes high turnover (osteitis fibrosa) and low turnover (adynamic bone disease) types.
- Diagnosis: Use of DEXA plus PTH, calcium, phosphate, and possibly bone biopsy.
- Treatment: Manage mineral metabolism, avoid high-risk medications like bisphosphonates in advanced CKD.

B. Chronic Liver Disease
- Hepatic osteodystrophy is common in cirrhosis, especially in alcohol-related liver disease.
- Impaired vitamin D metabolism and hypogonadism contribute.

- Management: Optimize liver function, supplement vitamin D and calcium, screen early.

Hematologic Disorders
A. Multiple Myeloma

- Bone lesions and fractures are common due to osteoclast activation.
- Screening: Serum protein electrophoresis (SPEP), urine Bence-Jones proteins.
- Treatment: Antimyeloma therapy, bisphosphonates (e.g., zoledronic acid), or denosumab.

B. Mastocytosis
- Systemic mast cell disorders can increase osteoclast activity.
- May present with fragility fractures and bone pain.
- Diagnosis: Bone marrow biopsy, tryptase levels.
- Management: Antihistamines, bisphosphonates, or interferon-alpha in severe cases.

RHEUMATOLOGIC AND AUTOIMMUNE DISEASES

A. Rheumatoid Arthritis (RA)

- Inflammation and glucocorticoid use lead to generalized and periarticular osteoporosis.
- Risk is high even in newly diagnosed RA patients.
- Management: Early disease control with DMARDs, minimize glucocorticoids, monitor BMD.

B. Systemic Lupus Erythematosus (SLE)

- Steroid use, renal disease, and vitamin D deficiency all contribute.
- Fracture risk is high, especially in young women.
- Treatment: Similar to RA; hydroxychloroquine may be bone-protective.

MEDICATION-INDUCED OSTEOPOROSIS

A. Glucocorticoids

- Among the most common causes of secondary osteoporosis.

- Risk increases with doses ≥5 mg/day for ≥3 months.
- Prevention: Start bisphosphonates and calcium/vitamin D early.

B. Anticonvulsants
- Enzyme inducers like phenytoin and carbamazepine reduce vitamin D levels.
- Management: Monitor vitamin D, consider alternative medications.

C. Aromatase Inhibitors
- Used in breast cancer, these agents reduce estrogen and increase bone loss.
- Intervention: BMD monitoring, bisphosphonates, and lifestyle modifications.

D. Proton Pump Inhibitors (PPIs)
- Long-term use may impair calcium absorption and increase fracture risk.
- Strategy: Use lowest effective dose; reassess long-term need.

E. SSRIs, Heparin, Methotrexate, and Chemotherapy
- Each can contribute to osteoporosis through various mechanisms.

- Management: Regular BMD monitoring and mitigation strategies depending on drug.

IMMOBILIZATION AND DISUSE SYNDROMES

- Prolonged bed rest, paralysis, and microgravity (e.g., spaceflight) reduce mechanical loading on bone.

- Leads to rapid bone loss, especially in lower extremities.
- Management: Mobilize early, use standing frames or neuromuscular electrical stimulation (NMES), consider pharmacologic therapy.

Genetic and Rare Disorders
A. Osteogenesis Imperfecta (OI)

- Genetic disorder causing brittle bones due to collagen defects.
- Present in children or adults depending on severity.
- Treatment: Bisphosphonates, orthopedic care, and rehabilitation.

B. Hypophosphatasia

- Rare metabolic bone disease caused by ALPL mutations.
- Characterized by fractures, dental loss, and poor mineralization.
- Diagnosis: Low serum alkaline phosphatase, genetic testing.
- Therapy: Enzyme replacement (asfotase alfa) in severe cases.

DIAGNOSTIC APPROACHES TO SUSPECTED OSTEOPOROSIS

A. Clinical Clues

- Young age (<50) with osteoporosis or fractures
- Unexpected low BMD in men
- Fractures despite normal BMD
- Refractory response to standard therapy

B. Laboratory Investigations

- Initial labs may include:
- CBC, ESR, CRP
- Serum calcium, phosphate, alkaline phosphatase
- 25(OH)D, PTH
- TSH, free T4

- Cortisol (AM or suppression test)
- Testosterone (men), estradiol (women)
- Creatinine, liver function tests
- SPEP/UPEP for myeloma screening

C. Imaging and Special Tests

- DEXA scan with vertebral fracture assessment
- X-rays for silent compression fractures
- Bone biopsy (rare, reserved for unclear cases)

TREATMENT PRINCIPLES

- Address the underlying cause as first-line therapy.
- Use anti-osteoporotic medications based on fracture risk, not just BMD.
- Avoid contraindicated drugs (e.g., bisphosphonates in severe CKD).
- Regular follow-up to monitor BMD, fracture risk, and treatment response.

Case Example

- Case: A 42-year-old man presents with low-trauma rib fractures. DEXA shows T-score of –2.8 at the lumbar spine. He has no family history of osteoporosis and leads a sedentary life.

Workup reveals:

- Low testosterone
- Elevated liver enzymes
- Positive celiac serology
- Diagnosis: Secondary osteoporosis due to undiagnosed celiac disease and hypogonadism.

Management:

- Gluten-free diet
- Endocrinology referral for testosterone therapy
- Calcium and vitamin D
- Consideration of bisphosphonate therapy

Secondary osteoporosis is a heterogeneous and underdiagnosed form of bone fragility. It is particularly prevalent in men, younger patients, and those with chronic illness or unusual fracture patterns. A systematic approach to evaluation, including detailed history, laboratory testing, and targeted imaging, is crucial. Proper identification and correction of the underlying cause, in conjunction with anti-osteoporotic therapy, can significantly reduce fracture risk and improve long-term outcomes.

CONCLUSION

Osteoporosis is a complex, multifactorial condition characterized by reduced bone mass and microarchitectural deterioration, leading to increased fracture risk. Its management requires a comprehensive, lifelong approach that extends beyond pharmacological treatment to encompass early detection, lifestyle interventions, patient education, and regular monitoring. As populations age globally, osteoporosis presents not only a clinical challenge but also a significant public health concern due to its burden on healthcare systems and its impact on patient quality of life.

Effective management begins with timely diagnosis, primarily through bone mineral density (BMD) assessments using DEXA scans, alongside fracture risk evaluation tools such as FRAX. Equally important is identifying secondary causes of osteoporosis, which allows for targeted therapy and improves outcomes. Non-pharmacological strategies — including calcium and vitamin D supplementation, weight-bearing exercise, smoking cessation, and fall prevention — form the cornerstone of prevention and treatment. These lifestyle modifications are particularly critical for older adults and individuals in high-risk or special populations, such as postmenopausal women, men with hypogonadism, and patients with comorbidities.

Pharmacological therapy has significantly evolved, with options ranging from antiresorptives like bisphosphonates and denosumab to anabolic agents such as teriparatide and romosozumab. Treatment decisions must be individualized based on patient risk profile, tolerance, fracture history, and response to therapy. Long-term success requires not only selecting the right drug but also addressing adherence, monitoring therapeutic efficacy, and making timely adjustments. Combination and sequential regimens are emerging as effective strategies to maximize bone strength and minimize fracture risk.

Tailored approaches are especially crucial for managing osteoporosis in special populations — including the elderly, those with renal impairment, or those with chronic steroid use — where treatment risks must be carefully balanced with benefits. Furthermore, the importance of multidisciplinary care, involving endocrinologists, geriatricians, physiotherapists, dietitians, and patient educators, cannot be overstated.

Looking forward, the future of osteoporosis management lies in precision medicine, regenerative therapies, digital health tools, and global initiatives aimed at improving awareness, early diagnosis, and continuity of care. With ongoing advancements in diagnostics, pharmacotherapy, and individualized care, osteoporosis is increasingly becoming a manageable chronic condition rather than an inevitable consequence of aging.

Ultimately, success in managing osteoporosis depends not only on medical innovation but also on proactive engagement by clinicians, caregivers, and patients alike — working together to preserve bone health, independence, and quality of life across the lifespan.

Printed in Dunstable, United Kingdom

77035462R00067